I0839484

WELCOME TO "MAXIMIZE YOUR MUSCLE: THE COMPREHENSIVE GUIDE TO OPTIMIZED WORKOUTS FOR MUSCLE GROWTH," A METICULOUSLY CURATED MANUAL DESIGNED TO TRANSFORM YOUR FITNESS JOURNEY BY MAXIMIZING YOUR POTENTIAL FOR MUSCULAR DEVELOPMENT. THIS BOOK IS NOT JUST A COLLECTION OF WORKOUTS; IT IS A HOLISTIC GUIDE PACKED WITH SCIENTIFICALLY PROVEN STRATEGIES, CUTTING-EDGE TRAINING TECHNIQUES, AND KEEN INSIGHTS AIMED AT PROMOTING MUSCLE GROWTH TO ITS UTMOST POTENTIAL.
IN TODAY'S FITNESS LANDSCAPE, WE ARE BOMBARDED BY COUNTLESS ADVICE, WORKOUT REGIMES, AND DIET PLANS THAT PROMISE RAPID MUSCLE GROWTH. WHILE SOME ARE EFFECTIVE, OTHERS MAY LEAD TO DISAPPOINTMENT, OR WORSE, INJURIES. IT'S A CHALLENGING AND CONFUSING PROCESS TO IDENTIFY WHICH METHODS WORK BEST FOR YOUR BODY TYPE, FITNESS LEVEL, AND LIFESTYLE.

THIS EBOOK WAS WRITTEN WITH A SINGLE, POWERFUL GOAL IN MIND: TO CUT THROUGH THE NOISE AND PROVIDE YOU WITH A SCIENCE-BASED, EFFECTIVE APPROACH TO MUSCLE BUILDING. HERE, WE UNDERSTAND THAT MUSCLE GROWTH IS NOT MERELY ABOUT LIFTING THE HEAVIEST WEIGHTS OR SPENDING ENDLESS HOURS AT THE GYM. INSTEAD, IT'S ABOUT UNDERSTANDING THE PHYSIOLOGY OF YOUR BODY, THE INTRICATE SCIENCE OF MUSCLE GROWTH, AND TAILORING A WORKOUT REGIME THAT RESPECTS THESE PRINCIPLES WHILE ALIGNING WITH YOUR PERSONAL GOALS AND CONSTRAINTS.

WE'LL START BY UNPACKING THE SCIENCE BEHIND MUSCLE GROWTH TO ESTABLISH A STRONG FOUNDATION FOR YOUR JOURNEY. FROM THE ROLES OF DIFFERENT MUSCLE FIBERS TO THE EFFECTS OF HORMONAL SHIFTS DURING WORKOUTS, WE WILL COVER IT ALL. FOLLOWING THIS, WE WILL DIVE INTO A DIVERSE ARRAY OF TRAINING PROGRAMS, EACH WITH DETAILED INSTRUCTIONS AND ILLUSTRATIONS. THEY ARE DESIGNED TO TARGET EVERY MAJOR MUSCLE GROUP IN YOUR BODY, ENSURING BALANCED AND PROPORTIONATE GROWTH.
ADDITIONALLY, WE WILL EXPLORE THE CRITICAL BUT OFTEN OVERLOOKED ASPECTS OF MUSCLE BUILDING: PROPER NUTRITION, RECOVERY, AND MINDSET. THESE ELEMENTS PLAY A VITAL ROLE IN OPTIMIZING YOUR WORKOUTS AND ACHIEVING SUSTAINABLE, LONG-TERM GROWTH. WITH THIS HOLISTIC VIEW, YOU WILL BE ABLE TO CRAFT A LIFESTYLE THAT SUPPORTS YOUR MUSCLE-BUILDING ASPIRATIONS.

WHETHER YOU ARE A BEGINNER STARTING ON YOUR JOURNEY, A SEASONED GYM-GOER STUCK IN A PLATEAU, OR A PROFESSIONAL BODYBUILDER LOOKING TO FINE-TUNE YOUR REGIMEN, THIS EBOOK IS YOUR INDISPENSABLE COMPANION. IT'S ABOUT TIME WE DISCARD THE ONE-SIZE-FITS-ALL APPROACH AND EMBRACE A METHOD THAT IS ROOTED IN SCIENTIFIC UNDERSTANDING AND PERSONALIZED FOR MAXIMUM EFFECTIVENESS.

AS YOU TURN THE PAGE, YOU ARE NOT MERELY READING A BOOK; YOU ARE BEGINNING A JOURNEY—A JOURNEY TO UNDERSTAND, TRAIN, AND TRANSFORM YOUR BODY LIKE NEVER BEFORE. SO GET READY TO EMBRACE THE SWEAT, ENDURE THE BURN, AND MOST IMPORTANTLY, WITNESS THE TRANSFORMATION THAT YOU'VE ALWAYS DREAMT OF.
WELCOME ABOARD TO A STRONGER, BIGGER, AND BETTER YOU. LET'S MAXIMIZE YOUR MUSCLE.

BELOW IS A SUMMARY OF KEY POINTS WE'LL BE GOING OVER IN THIS BOOK:

CHAPTER 1: UNDERSTANDING THE SCIENCE OF MUSCLE GROWTH

IN THIS CHAPTER, WE UNRAVEL THE SCIENCE BEHIND MUSCLE GROWTH, WHICH IS PIVOTAL TO CREATING EFFECTIVE WORKOUT ROUTINES. WE'LL DISCUSS WHAT HAPPENS TO YOUR MUSCLES DURING A WORKOUT, THE ROLE OF MUSCLE FIBERS, THE IMPACT OF HORMONES, AND HOW YOUR BODY REPAIRS AND GROWS MUSCLES.

CHAPTER 2: THE ROLE OF NUTRITION IN MUSCLE GROWTH

THIS CHAPTER UNDERLINES THE IMPORTANCE OF A BALANCED DIET IN MUSCLE BUILDING. WE DELVE INTO THE MACRO AND MICRONUTRIENTS ESSENTIAL FOR MUSCLE GROWTH, THE BEST SOURCES OF THESE NUTRIENTS, AND THE OPTIMAL TIMES TO CONSUME THEM. WE ALSO DISCUSS THE ROLE OF SUPPLEMENTS AND HOW TO INCORPORATE THEM WISELY INTO YOUR DIET.

CHAPTER 3: DESIGNING A MUSCLE-BUILDING WORKOUT REGIME

HERE, WE PROVIDE YOU WITH A GUIDE TO CRAFTING YOUR PERSONALIZED MUSCLE-BUILDING WORKOUT ROUTINE. WE'LL COVER THE KEY COMPONENTS OF AN EFFECTIVE WORKOUT, PRINCIPLES OF WEIGHT LIFTING, AND TIPS ON BALANCING DIFFERENT MUSCLE GROUPS TO CREATE A COMPREHENSIVE AND BALANCED FITNESS PLAN.

CHAPTER 4: WORKOUT PROGRAMS FOR MAXIMUM MUSCLE GROWTH

IN THIS CHAPTER, YOU'LL FIND A SELECTION OF DETAILED WORKOUT PROGRAMS, EACH TARGETING DIFFERENT MUSCLE GROUPS AND FITNESS LEVELS. FROM BEGINNER TO ADVANCED, THESE PROGRAMS WILL PROVIDE YOU WITH THE TOOLS TO PUSH YOUR BODY TO NEW HEIGHTS AND WITNESS MAXIMUM MUSCLE GROWTH.

CHAPTER 5: RECOVERY: THE OVERLOOKED COMPONENT OF MUSCLE GROWTH

THIS CHAPTER HIGHLIGHTS THE CRITICAL ROLE OF REST AND RECOVERY IN MUSCLE GROWTH. WE WILL DISCUSS THE IMPORTANCE OF SLEEP, ACTIVE RECOVERY DAYS, AND STRETCHING, PROVIDING PRACTICAL TIPS ON HOW TO INCORPORATE THESE ELEMENTS INTO YOUR ROUTINE TO OPTIMIZE MUSCLE REPAIR AND GROWTH.

CHAPTER 6: MENTAL TOUGHNESS AND CONSISTENCY: THE KEY TO SUSTAINABLE GROWTH

IN THIS CHAPTER, WE EMPHASIZE THE IMPORTANCE OF MENTAL FORTITUDE AND CONSISTENCY IN YOUR MUSCLE GROWTH JOURNEY. WE'LL SHARE TECHNIQUES TO STAY MOTIVATED, OVERCOME PLATEAUS, AND KEEP PROGRESSING TOWARDS YOUR FITNESS GOALS.

CHAPTER 7: THE ROLE OF NUTRITION FOR MAXIMIZING MUSCLE GROWTH

THE JOURNEY TO MUSCLE GROWTH ISN'T CONFINED TO THE HOURS SPENT LIFTING WEIGHTS IN THE GYM. WHILE THE RIGHT TRAINING REGIMEN IS CRUCIAL, PROPER NUTRITION CAN SIGNIFICANTLY ENHANCE MUSCLE GROWTH, RECOVERY, AND OVERALL PHYSICAL PERFORMANCE. THIS CHAPTER EXPLORES THE VITAL ROLE OF NUTRITION IN MUSCLE GROWTH AND OFFERS GUIDELINES FOR FUELING YOUR BODY EFFECTIVELY FOR MAXIMUM GAINS.

CONCLUSION

WE'LL WRAP UP WITH A RECAP OF THE KEY POINTS COVERED IN THIS EBOOK AND PROVIDE SOME FINAL THOUGHTS TO KEEP IN MIND AS YOU EMBARK ON YOUR JOURNEY TOWARDS MAXIMUM MUSCLE GROWTH.

CHAPTER 1: UNDERSTANDING THE SCIENCE OF MUSCLE GROWTH

UNDERSTANDING THE SCIENCE OF MUSCLE GROWTH IS FUNDAMENTAL TO ACHIEVING YOUR MUSCLE-BUILDING GOALS. IT ALLOWS US TO DESIGN EFFECTIVE WORKOUT PROGRAMS, UNDERSTAND THE ROLE OF NUTRITION, AND APPRECIATE THE IMPORTANCE OF RECOVERY. IN THIS CHAPTER, WE'LL DELVE INTO THE BASICS OF MUSCLE PHYSIOLOGY AND GROWTH.

SECTION 1.1: THE BASICS OF MUSCLE PHYSIOLOGY

THE HUMAN BODY COMPRISES OVER 600 MUSCLES, EACH PLAYING A VITAL ROLE IN MAINTAINING OUR BODY'S FUNCTIONALITY. THESE MUSCLES ARE MADE UP OF INDIVIDUAL MUSCLE FIBERS THAT BUNDLE TOGETHER TO FORM A SINGLE MUSCLE. THERE ARE TWO MAIN TYPES OF MUSCLE FIBERS:

1. TYPE I (SLOW TWITCH) FIBERS: THESE FIBERS HAVE A HIGH CAPACITY FOR OXYGEN USE AND ARE FATIGUERESISTANT, MAKING THEM IDEAL FOR ENDURANCE ACTIVITIES LIKE DISTANCE RUNNING.

2. TYPE II (FAST TWITCH) FIBERS: THESE FIBERS FATIGUE FASTER BUT ARE CAPABLE OF MORE POWERFUL, SHORT DURATION MOVEMENTS, SUCH AS WEIGHTLIFTING OR SPRINTING. UNDERSTANDING THESE FIBER TYPES IS CRUCIAL AS DIFFERENT EXERCISES CAN STIMULATE AND DEVELOP DIFFERENT TYPES OF FIBERS, AFFECTING YOUR MUSCLE GROWTH AND PHYSIQUE.

SECTION 1.2: WHAT HAPPENS TO YOUR MUSCLES DURING A WORKOUT

WHEN YOU LIFT WEIGHTS OR PERFORM RESISTANCE EXERCISES, YOU CREATE MICRO-TEARS IN YOUR MUSCLE FIBERS, PARTICULARLY IN THE FAST-TWITCH TYPE. THIS PROCESS IS KNOWN AS 'MUSCLE PROTEIN BREAKDOWN' (MPB). THOUGH IT MIGHT SOUND DETRIMENTAL, THIS PROCESS IS THE FIRST STEP TOWARD MUSCLE GROWTH.

SECTION 1.3: THE PROCESS OF MUSCLE GROWTH (HYPERTROPHY)

MUSCLE GROWTH, OR HYPERTROPHY, OCCURS DURING THE RECOVERY PERIOD AFTER THE WORKOUT. YOUR BODY REPAIRS THE DAMAGED MUSCLE FIBERS THROUGH A CELLULAR PROCESS WHERE IT FUSES MUSCLE FIBERS TOGETHER TO FORM NEW MUSCLE PROTEIN STRANDS OR MYOFIBRILS. THESE REPAIRED MYOFIBRILS INCREASE IN THICKNESS AND NUMBER TO CREATE MUSCLE HYPERTROPHY (GROWTH). THIS GROWTH PROCESS IS FUELED BY THE PROTEINS YOU CONSUME. PROTEIN SYNTHESIS MUST EXCEED PROTEIN BREAKDOWN (THE MPB MENTIONED EARLIER) FOR MUSCLE GROWTH TO OCCUR. THAT'S WHY ADEQUATE PROTEIN INTAKE AND RECOVERY ARE CRITICAL COMPONENTS OF MUSCLE GROWTH, WHICH WE'LL EXPLORE IN SUBSEQUENT CHAPTERS.

SECTION 1.4: HORMONES AND MUSCLE GROWTH

HORMONES PLAY A VITAL ROLE IN MUSCLE GROWTH. THE MOST CRITICAL ARE:
1. TESTOSTERONE: THIS HORMONE PROMOTES MUSCLE GROWTH BY STIMULATING PROTEIN SYNTHESIS, INHIBITING PROTEIN BREAKDOWN, AND ACTIVATING SATELLITE CELLS (CELLS INVOLVED IN MUSCLE REPAIR AND REGENERATION).

2. GROWTH HORMONE (GH):

GH AIDS IN MUSCLE GROWTH BY STIMULATING PROTEIN SYNTHESIS, INTERACTING WITH INSULIN-LIKE GROWTH FACTOR (IGF-1) TO PROMOTE MUSCLE CELL PRODUCTION, AND ENHANCING THE BODY'S USE OF FAT FOR ENERGY.

3. INSULIN-LIKE GROWTH FACTOR (IGF-1):

PRODUCED IN THE LIVER AND MUSCLE CELLS, IGF-1 WORKS WITH GH TO PROMOTE AMINO ACID UPTAKE AND PROTEIN SYNTHESIS IN MUSCLE CELLS. UNDERSTANDING THESE HORMONAL INFLUENCES CAN HELP OPTIMIZE YOUR WORKOUT AND NUTRITION PLAN TO ENHANCE MUSCLE GROWTH.

SECTION 1.5: ADAPTATION AND PROGRESSIVE OVERLOAD

FINALLY, REMEMBER THAT OUR BODIES ARE INCREDIBLY ADAPTIVE. WHAT INITIALLY CAUSES MUSCLE DAMAGE AND SUBSEQUENT GROWTH WON'T CONTINUE TO DO SO INDEFINITELY. THIS CONCEPT IS WHERE THE PRINCIPLE OF PROGRESSIVE OVERLOAD COMES IN: TO CONTINUE GROWING, MUSCLES NEED TO BE SUBJECTED TO INCREASING LEVELS OF STRESS OVER TIME.

IN THE FOLLOWING CHAPTERS, WE WILL DISCUSS HOW TO USE THE PRINCIPLE OF PROGRESSIVE OVERLOAD IN YOUR TRAINING REGIMEN, THE CRITICAL ROLE OF NUTRITION, AND THE OFTEN OVERLOOKED ASPECT OF RECOVERY. THIS KNOWLEDGE, GROUNDED IN THE SCIENCE OF MUSCLE GROWTH, WILL EQUIP YOU TO MAXIMIZE YOUR WORKOUTS AND REALIZE YOUR MUSCLE-BUILDING POTENTIAL. TO TRULY MAXIMIZE MUSCLE GROWTH, IT'S ESSENTIAL TO GRASP THESE FUNDAMENTAL PRINCIPLES. BY UNDERSTANDING THE BIOLOGY BEHIND THE PROCESS, YOU CAN MAKE MORE INFORMED DECISIONS ABOUT YOUR WORKOUT ROUTINES, NUTRITION, AND RECOVERY STRATEGIES, AND ULTIMATELY ACHIEVE YOUR MUSCLE-BUILDING GOALS MORE EFFECTIVELY.

CHAPTER 2: THE ROLE OF NUTRITION IN MUSCLE GROWTH

THE SAYING "YOU ARE WHAT YOU EAT" IS PARTICULARLY RELEVANT WHEN IT COMES TO MUSCLE GROWTH. WHILE WORKOUTS TRIGGER THE PROCESS OF MUSCLE DEVELOPMENT, NUTRITION PROVIDES THE BUILDING BLOCKS NECESSARY FOR THIS GROWTH. IN THIS CHAPTER, WE'LL EXPLORE THE CRUCIAL ROLE OF NUTRITION IN MUSCLE GROWTH AND PROVIDE GUIDANCE ON WHAT, WHEN, AND HOW MUCH TO EAT.

SECTION 2.1: THE IMPORTANCE OF MACRONUTRIENTS

MACRONUTRIENTS ARE THE NUTRIENTS YOUR BODY NEEDS IN LARGE AMOUNTS TO FUNCTION CORRECTLY, NAMELY CARBOHYDRATES, PROTEINS, AND FATS. EACH OF THESE MACRONUTRIENTS PLAYS A VITAL ROLE IN MUSCLE GROWTH.

1. PROTEINS: PROTEINS ARE THE BUILDING BLOCKS OF MUSCLE TISSUE. THEY ARE ESSENTIAL FOR REPAIRING THE MICRO-TEARS IN MUSCLE FIBERS CAUSED BY INTENSE WORKOUTS, LEADING TO MUSCLE GROWTH. AIM TO CONSUME A SUFFICIENT AMOUNT OF PROTEIN THROUGHOUT THE DAY, PARTICULARLY AFTER YOUR WORKOUTS, TO SUPPORT THIS GROWTH.

2. CARBOHYDRATES: CARBS ARE THE PRIMARY SOURCE OF ENERGY FOR YOUR WORKOUTS. THEY FUEL YOUR MUSCLES DURING EXERCISE AND REPLENISH GLYCOGEN STORES AFTERWARD. CONSUMING CARBS POST-WORKOUT CAN ALSO SPIKE INSULIN LEVELS, WHICH HELPS DECREASE PROTEIN BREAKDOWN AND PROMOTE MUSCLE RECOVERY AND GROWTH.

3. FATS: HEALTHY FATS PLAY A CRUCIAL ROLE IN HORMONE PRODUCTION, INCLUDING TESTOSTERONE AND GROWTH HORMONES THAT ARE ESSENTIAL FOR MUSCLE GROWTH. ADDITIONALLY, FATS PROVIDE A RICH SOURCE OF CALORIES, BENEFICIAL IF YOU'RE LOOKING TO INCREASE MUSCLE MASS.

SECTION 2.2: THE ROLE OF MICRONUTRIENTS

MICRONUTRIENTS, INCLUDING VITAMINS AND MINERALS, ARE REQUIRED IN SMALLER AMOUNTS BUT ARE STILL CRITICAL TO MUSCLE GROWTH AND OVERALL HEALTH. FOR INSTANCE, VITAMIN D IS ESSENTIAL FOR BONE HEALTH AND MUSCLE FUNCTION, WHILE MINERALS LIKE CALCIUM AND MAGNESIUM PLAY A CRUCIAL ROLE IN MUSCLE CONTRACTION AND RELAXATION.

SECTION 2.3: HYDRATION

WATER IS ESSENTIAL FOR NEARLY EVERY BODILY FUNCTION, INCLUDING NUTRIENT TRANSPORT AND MUSCLE RECOVERY. STAYING PROPERLY HYDRATED NOT ONLY HELPS YOU PERFORM YOUR BEST DURING WORKOUTS BUT ALSO SUPPORTS OPTIMAL MUSCLE RECOVERY AND GROWTH.

SECTION 2.4: NUTRIENT TIMING

WHEN YOU EAT CAN BE JUST AS IMPORTANT AS WHAT YOU EAT WHEN IT COMES TO MUSCLE GROWTH. CONSUMING A BALANCED MIX OF PROTEINS AND CARBOHYDRATES POST-WORKOUT CAN OPTIMIZE MUSCLE PROTEIN SYNTHESIS AND PROMOTE RECOVERY. ADDITIONALLY, REGULAR PROTEIN INTAKE THROUGHOUT THE DAY CAN ENSURE A CONSTANT SUPPLY OF AMINO ACIDS FOR ONGOING MUSCLE REPAIR AND GROWTH.

SECTION 2.5: SUPPLEMENTS FOR MUSCLE GROWTH

WHILE A BALANCED, WHOLE-FOOD DIET SHOULD ALWAYS BE YOUR PRIMARY SOURCE OF NUTRIENTS, CERTAIN SUPPLEMENTS CAN SUPPORT MUSCLE GROWTH. PROTEIN POWDERS, CREATINE, AND BRANCHED-CHAIN AMINO ACIDS (BCAAS) ARE COMMONLY USED SUPPLEMENTS IN THE MUSCLE-BUILDING WORLD. HOWEVER, ALWAYS CONSULT WITH A HEALTHCARE PROFESSIONAL BEFORE STARTING ANY SUPPLEMENT REGIMEN.

SECTION 2.6: CUSTOMIZING YOUR NUTRITION FOR MUSCLE GROWTH

NUTRITION NEEDS CAN VARY WIDELY DEPENDING ON INDIVIDUAL FACTORS SUCH AS AGE, SEX, BODY COMPOSITION, ACTIVITY LEVEL, AND FITNESS GOALS. IT'S CRUCIAL TO PERSONALIZE YOUR NUTRITION PLAN TO YOUR NEEDS. A REGISTERED DIETITIAN OR CERTIFIED NUTRITIONIST CAN PROVIDE VALUABLE GUIDANCE HERE. IN CONCLUSION, A WELL-PLANNED NUTRITION STRATEGY IS CRUCIAL FOR MAXIMIZING MUSCLE GROWTH. BY UNDERSTANDING THE ROLES OF MACRONUTRIENTS, MICRONUTRIENTS, HYDRATION, NUTRIENT TIMING, AND SUPPLEMENTS, YOU CAN CREATE A NUTRITION PLAN TAILORED TO YOUR MUSCLE GROWTH GOALS. HOWEVER, REMEMBER THAT NUTRITION IS JUST ONE PIECE OF THE PUZZLE, COMPLEMENTING YOUR WORKOUT AND RECOVERY STRATEGIES, WHICH WE'LL EXPLORE IN THE FOLLOWING CHAPTERS.

CHAPTER 3: DESIGNING A MUSCLE-BUILDING WORKOUT REGIME

CREATING A MUSCLE-BUILDING WORKOUT ROUTINE THAT IS EFFICIENT, SAFE, AND TAILORED TO YOUR SPECIFIC GOALS IS PIVOTAL TO MAXIMIZING MUSCLE GROWTH. IN THIS CHAPTER, WE'LL EXPLORE THE ESSENTIAL ELEMENTS OF SUCH A ROUTINE, PROVIDE GUIDANCE ON CREATING YOUR PERSONALIZED REGIMEN, AND DISCUSS SOME KEY PRINCIPLES TO KEEP IN MIND.

SECTION 3.1: ESSENTIAL COMPONENTS OF A MUSCLE-BUILDING WORKOUT

THE KEY ELEMENTS TO CONSIDER WHEN CREATING A MUSCLE-BUILDING WORKOUT INCLUDE:

1. EXERCISE SELECTION: PRIORITIZE COMPOUND MOVEMENTS THAT ENGAGE MULTIPLE MUSCLE GROUPS SIMULTANEOUSLY, SUCH AS SQUATS, DEADLIFTS, AND BENCH PRESSES. THESE EXERCISES STIMULATE A GREATER HORMONAL RESPONSE AND ALLOW FOR MORE SIGNIFICANT MUSCLE GROWTH OVERALL.

2. VOLUME: VOLUME (SETS X REPS X WEIGHT) IS A CRUCIAL FACTOR FOR HYPERTROPHY. HOWEVER, IT'S ESSENTIAL TO STRIKE A BALANCE; TOO LITTLE VOLUME CAN LIMIT GROWTH, WHILE TOO MUCH CAN LEAD TO OVERTRAINING AND INJURIES.

3. INTENSITY: LIFTING HEAVIER WEIGHTS (AROUND 70-85% OF YOUR ONE-REPETITION MAXIMUM) TYPICALLY PROMOTES MUSCLE GROWTH BY EFFECTIVELY STIMULATING YOUR MUSCLES.

4. FREQUENCY: TRAINING FREQUENCY REFERS TO HOW OFTEN YOU TRAIN EACH MUSCLE GROUP. RESEARCH SUGGESTS TRAINING EACH MUSCLE GROUP AT LEAST TWO TIMES PER WEEK FOR OPTIMAL GROWTH.

SECTION 3.2: STRUCTURING YOUR WORKOUT PLAN

HERE'S A GENERAL GUIDELINE ON HOW TO STRUCTURE YOUR MUSCLE-BUILDING WORKOUT PLAN:

1. WARM-UP: ALWAYS START WITH A WARM-UP TO PREPARE YOUR MUSCLES AND JOINTS FOR THE WORKOUT. THIS STEP COULD INCLUDE LIGHT CARDIO AND DYNAMIC STRETCHING.

2. STRENGTH TRAINING: AFTER WARMING UP, MOVE ONTO YOUR STRENGTH TRAINING EXERCISES. REMEMBER TO BALANCE YOUR WORKOUTS TO TRAIN ALL MAJOR MUSCLE GROUPS EVENLY OVER THE WEEK.

3. COOL-DOWN: FINISH WITH A COOL-DOWN PHASE, INCLUDING LIGHTER ACTIVITIES AND STRETCHING TO HELP START THE RECOVERY PROCESS.

SECTION 3.3: THE IMPORTANCE OF PROGRESSIVE OVERLOAD

PROGRESSIVE OVERLOAD, OR GRADUALLY INCREASING THE STRESS PLACED ON YOUR BODY DURING WORKOUTS, IS VITAL TO CONTINUAL MUSCLE GROWTH. THIS PRINCIPLE CAN BE APPLIED BY INCREASING THE WEIGHT LIFTED, THE VOLUME OF WORK DONE, OR THE INTENSITY OF EXERCISES OVER TIME.

SECTION 3.4: BALANCING WORKOUTS

IT'S CRUCIAL TO MAINTAIN A BALANCED WORKOUT PLAN THAT ADEQUATELY TARGETS ALL MUSCLE GROUPS TO PREVENT IMBALANCES AND INJURIES. A WELL-ROUNDED PLAN SHOULD INVOLVE EXERCISES FOR YOUR UPPER BODY, LOWER BODY, AND CORE.

SECTION 3.5: REST AND RECOVERY

INCORPORATE REST DAYS INTO YOUR WORKOUT SCHEDULE TO ALLOW FOR MUSCLE RECOVERY AND GROWTH. OVERTRAINING CAN LEAD TO EXCESSIVE MUSCLE BREAKDOWN, IMPAIRING YOUR MUSCLE GROWTH AND INCREASING INJURY RISK.

SECTION 3.6: LISTEN TO YOUR BODY

WHILE PUSHING YOUR LIMITS IS PART OF THE PROCESS, IT'S EQUALLY IMPORTANT TO LISTEN TO YOUR BODY. IF YOU'RE FEELING OVERLY FATIGUED, EXPERIENCING PAIN DURING A WORKOUT, OR NOT RECOVERING WELL, THESE ARE SIGNS THAT YOU MAY NEED TO ADJUST YOUR ROUTINE. IN THE FOLLOWING CHAPTER, WE WILL DELVE INTO A SELECTION OF SPECIFIC WORKOUT PROGRAMS THAT INCORPORATE THESE PRINCIPLES AND CAN BE TAILORED TO VARIOUS FITNESS LEVELS AND MUSCLE GROWTH GOALS. REMEMBER, CONSISTENCY IS KEY IN ANY WORKOUT REGIMEN, AND IT'S A MARATHON, NOT A SPRINT. YOUR MUSCLE-BUILDING JOURNEY IS UNIQUE TO YOU, SO CREATE AND ADJUST YOUR PLAN ACCORDING TO WHAT SUITS YOU BEST AND HELPS YOU REACH YOUR GOALS SAFELY AND EFFECTIVELY.

BELOW ARE EXAMPLES OF MUSCLE-BUILDING EXERCISES CATEGORIZED BY THE MAJOR MUSCLE GROUPS THEY TARGET: ALL EXERCISES ARE ILLUSTRATED AT THE REAR SECTION OF THE BOOK.

1. LEGS & GLUTES

• SQUATS: THIS COMPOUND EXERCISE TARGETS YOUR QUADRICEPS, HAMSTRINGS, AND GLUTES. IT ALSO RECRUITS YOUR CORE MUSCLES.
• DEADLIFTS: DEADLIFTS WORK YOUR ENTIRE LOWER BODY, PARTICULARLY YOUR HAMSTRINGS AND GLUTES, AND ALSO ENGAGE YOUR LOWER BACK AND CORE.
• LUNGES: THIS EXERCISE PRIMARILY TARGETS YOUR QUADRICEPS BUT ALSO WORKS YOUR HAMSTRINGS, GLUTES, AND CALVES.
• LEG PRESS: THE LEG PRESS IS AN EXCELLENT EXERCISE FOR TARGETING THE QUADRICEPS, HAMSTRINGS, AND GLUTES.

2. CHEST

• BENCH PRESS: THIS COMPOUND MOVEMENT PRIMARILY TARGETS THE PECTORAL (CHEST) MUSCLES AND ALSO RECRUITS THE TRICEPS AND SHOULDERS.
• INCLINE/DECLINE BENCH PRESS: VARIATIONS OF THE BENCH PRESS THAT TARGET DIFFERENT PORTIONS OF THE CHEST MUSCLES.
• DUMBBELL FLYES: THIS EXERCISE ISOLATES THE CHEST MUSCLES.

3. BACK

• PULL-UPS: PULL-UPS ARE A GREAT COMPOUND EXERCISE THAT WORKS THE ENTIRE BACK, PARTICULARLY THE LATISSIMUS DORSI, AS WELL AS THE BICEPS.
• BENT-OVER ROWS: THIS EXERCISE TARGETS THE BACK MUSCLES, INCLUDING THE LATS AND RHOMBOIDS.
• LAT PULLDOWNS: THIS EXERCISE PRIMARILY TARGETS THE LATS.

4. SHOULDERS
• OVERHEAD PRESS (BARBELL OR DUMBBELL): THIS COMPOUND EXERCISE PRIMARILY TARGETS THE DELTOIDS IN
THE SHOULDERS AND ALSO WORKS THE TRICEPS.
• LATERAL RAISES: THIS EXERCISE ISOLATES THE LATERAL (SIDE) DELTOIDS.
• FRONT RAISES: THIS EXERCISE ISOLATES THE ANTERIOR (FRONT) DELTOIDS.

5. ARMS
• BICEP CURLS (BARBELL OR DUMBBELL): THIS EXERCISE TARGETS THE BICEPS.
• TRICEP PUSHDOWNS: THIS EXERCISE ISOLATES THE TRICEPS.
• HAMMER CURLS: THIS EXERCISE WORKS THE BICEPS AND THE BRACHIALIS, A MUSCLE OF THE UPPER ARM

6. CORE
• PLANKS: THIS EXERCISE TARGETS THE ENTIRE CORE AND ALSO PROMOTES STABILITY AND BALANCE.
• RUSSIAN TWISTS: THIS EXERCISE WORKS THE OBLIQUES.
• LEG RAISES: THIS EXERCISE TARGETS THE LOWER ABDOMINALS.

REMEMBER, PROPER FORM AND TECHNIQUE ARE CRITICAL WHEN PERFORMING THESE EXERCISES TO EFFECTIVELY TARGET THE RIGHT MUSCLES AND PREVENT INJURY. IT'S ALWAYS A GOOD IDEA TO SEEK THE GUIDANCE OF A FITNESS PROFESSIONAL WHEN STARTING A NEW WORKOUT REGIMEN OR LEARNING NEW EXERCISES.

CHAPTER 4: WORKOUT PROGRAMS FOR MAXIMUM MUSCLE GROWTH

NOW THAT WE UNDERSTAND THE SCIENCE BEHIND MUSCLE GROWTH AND THE PRINCIPLES OF DESIGNING A WORKOUT ROUTINE, LET'S DELVE INTO SPECIFIC WORKOUT PROGRAMS. EACH PROGRAM IS DESIGNED TO CATER TO DIFFERENT FITNESS LEVELS AND GOALS. REMEMBER TO CONSULT WITH A FITNESS PROFESSIONAL TO ENSURE THESE PROGRAMS ALIGN WITH YOUR INDIVIDUAL NEEDS AND CAPACITIES.

SECTION 4.1: BEGINNER'S PROGRAM

IF YOU'RE NEW TO STRENGTH TRAINING, IT'S CRUCIAL TO START WITH A PROGRAM THAT INTRODUCES YOU TO THE BASICS. THIS BEGINNER'S PROGRAM FOCUSES ON COMPOUND MOVEMENTS TO ENGAGE MULTIPLE MUSCLE GROUPS SIMULTANEOUSLY AND BUILD A SOLID STRENGTH FOUNDATION. ALL EXERCISES ARE ILLUSTRATED AT THE REAR SECTION OF THE BOOK.

DAY 1 – FULL BODY WORKOUT:
• SQUATS: 3 SETS OF 10-12 REPS
• BENCH PRESS: 3 SETS OF 10-12 REPS
• BENT-OVER ROWS: 3 SETS OF 10-12 REPS
• OVERHEAD PRESS: 2 SETS OF 10-12 REPS
• DEADLIFTS: 2 SETS OF 10-12 REPS
REST FOR AT LEAST ONE DAY BETWEEN EACH WORKOUT DAY, FOCUSING ON ACTIVE RECOVERY AND FLEXIBILITY.

SECTION 4.2: INTERMEDIATE PROGRAM

AFTER A FEW MONTHS OF CONSISTENT TRAINING, YOU MAY BE READY FOR AN INTERMEDIATE PROGRAM. THIS SPLIT ROUTINE ALLOWS FOR A HIGHER VOLUME PER MUSCLE GROUP AND ADEQUATE RECOVERY TIME.

DAY 1 – CHEST AND TRICEPS:
• BENCH PRESS: 4 SETS OF 8-10 REPS
• INCLINE DUMBBELL PRESS: 3 SETS OF 8-10 REPS
• DUMBBELL FLYES: 3 SETS OF 10-12 REPS
• TRICEP PUSHDOWNS: 3 SETS OF 10-12 REPS
• SKULL CRUSHERS: 3 SETS OF 10-12 REPS

DAY 2 – BACK AND BICEPS:
• DEADLIFTS: 4 SETS OF 8-10 REPS
• PULL-UPS: 3 SETS OF 10 REPS (OR TO FAILURE)
• BENT-OVER ROWS: 3 SETS OF 8-10 REPS
• BICEP CURLS: 3 SETS OF 10-12 REPS
• HAMMER CURLS: 3 SETS OF 10-12 REPS

DAY 3 – LEGS AND SHOULDERS:
• SQUATS: 4 SETS OF 8-10 REPS
• LUNGES: 3 SETS OF 10 REPS (EACH LEG)
• CALF RAISES: 3 SETS OF 15 REPS
• OVERHEAD PRESS: 3 SETS OF 8-10 REPS
• LATERAL RAISES: 3 SETS OF 10-12 REPS

IMPLEMENT THIS ROUTINE ON NON-CONSECUTIVE DAYS (E.G., MONDAY, WEDNESDAY, FRIDAY) TO ALLOW FOR ADEQUATE

SECTION 4.3: ADVANCED PROGRAM
THIS ADVANCED PROGRAM INTRODUCES A HIGHER VOLUME AND VARIETY OF EXERCISES, FOCUSING ON INDIVIDUAL MUSCLE GROUPS EACH DAY FOR MAXIMUM MUSCLE STIMULATION.

DAY 1 - CHEST:
- BENCH PRESS: 5 SETS OF 5 REPS
- INCLINE DUMBBELL PRESS: 4 SETS OF 8 REPS
- DUMBBELL FLYES: 3 SETS OF 10 REPS
- CABLE CROSSOVERS: 3 SETS OF 12 REPS

DAY 2 - BACK:
- DEADLIFTS: 5 SETS OF 5 REPS
- PULL-UPS: 4 SETS TO FAILURE
- BENT-OVER ROWS: 4 SETS OF 8 REPS
- LAT PULLDOWNS: 3 SETS OF 10 REPS

DAY 3 - LEGS:
- SQUATS: 5 SETS OF 5 REPS
- LUNGES: 4 SETS OF 10 REPS (EACH LEG)
- LEG PRESS: 4 SETS OF 8 REPS
- CALF RAISES: 3 SETS OF 15 REPS

DAY 4 - SHOULDERS:
- OVERHEAD PRESS: 5 SETS OF 5 REPS
- LATERAL RAISES: 3 SETS OF 10 REPS
- FRONT RAISES: 3 SETS OF 10 REPS
- REAR DELT FLYES: 3 SETS OF 10 REPS

DAY 5 - ARMS:
- BICEP CURLS: 4 SETS OF 8 REPS
- HAMMER CURLS: 3 SETS OF 10 REPS
- TRICEP PUSHDOWNS: 4 SETS OF 8 REPS
- SKULL CRUSHERS: 3 SETS OF 10 REPS

FOR THIS PROGRAM, ENSURE YOU'RE TAKING AT LEAST ONE REST DAY AFTER EACH TRAINING DAY (E.G., TRAIN ON MONDAY,WEDNESDAY, FRIDAY, SUNDAY, TUESDAY) AND ADJUST AS NEEDED FOR RECOVERY. THESE WORKOUT PROGRAMS PROVIDE A STRUCTURED APPROACH TO MUSCLE GROWTH, FROM BEGINNER TO ADVANCED. REMEMBER, HOWEVER, THAT THE EFFECTIVENESS OF THESE PROGRAMS HINGES ON PROPER FORM, CONSISTENCY, AND COUPLING THEM WITH APPROPRIATE NUTRITION AND RECOVERY PRACTICES. ALWAYS LISTEN TO YOUR BODY AND ADJUST YOUR REGIMEN AS NEEDED TO STAY HEALTHY AND KEEP MAKING PROGRESS TOWARDS YOUR MUSCLE GROWTH GOALS.

CHAPTER 5: RECOVERY: THE OVERLOOKED COMPONENT OF MUSCLE GROWTH

RECOVERY OFTEN GETS SIDELINED IN DISCUSSIONS AROUND MUSCLE GROWTH, BUT IT'S ONE OF THE MOST CRITICAL COMPONENTS OF THE PROCESS. EXERCISE INITIATES MUSCLE GROWTH, BUT THE ACTUAL GROWTH HAPPENS DURING RECOVERY. IN THIS CHAPTER, WE WILL EXPLORE THE IMPORTANCE OF RECOVERY AND PROVIDE PRACTICAL STRATEGIES TO ENHANCE YOUR RECOVERY PROCESS.

SECTION 5.1: THE IMPORTANCE OF RECOVERY IN MUSCLE GROWTH

DURING A WORKOUT, YOUR MUSCLES UNDERGO STRESS, CAUSING MICRO-TEARS IN THE MUSCLE FIBERS. DURING RECOVERY, YOUR BODY REPAIRS THESE DAMAGED MUSCLE TISSUES, LEADING TO MUSCLE GROWTH. IF RECOVERY IS INSUFFICIENT, THE MUSCLE TISSUES CAN'T REPAIR EFFECTIVELY, HINDERING YOUR MUSCLE GROWTH AND INCREASING YOUR RISK OF INJURIES.

SECTION 5.2: QUALITY SLEEP FOR RECOVERY

SLEEP IS THE MOST POWERFUL RECOVERY TOOL AT YOUR DISPOSAL. DURING SLEEP, YOUR BODY PRODUCES GROWTH HORMONE, WHICH IS CRUCIAL FOR MUSCLE REPAIR AND GROWTH. AIM FOR 7-9 HOURS OF QUALITY SLEEP PER NIGHT TO SUPPORT OPTIMAL MUSCLE RECOVERY.

SECTION 5.3: ACTIVE RECOVERY

ACTIVE RECOVERY INVOLVES LIGHT, LOW-INTENSITY ACTIVITIES ON YOUR REST DAYS. IT PROMOTES BLOOD CIRCULATION, HELPING DELIVER NUTRIENTS TO YOUR MUSCLES TO AID RECOVERY. EXAMPLES OF ACTIVE RECOVERY ACTIVITIES INCLUDE WALKING, LIGHT CYCLING, AND YOGA.

SECTION 5.4: NUTRITION AND HYDRATION FOR RECOVERY

AS COVERED IN CHAPTER 2, NUTRITION PLAYS A CRUCIAL ROLE IN RECOVERY. CONSUMING A MEAL RICH IN PROTEIN AND CARBOHYDRATES WITHIN A COUPLE OF HOURS AFTER YOUR WORKOUT CAN MAXIMIZE MUSCLE PROTEIN SYNTHESIS. HYDRATION IS ALSO VITAL AS IT AIDS IN NUTRIENT TRANSPORT AND MUSCLE FUNCTION.

SECTION 5.5: REST DAYS

REST DAYS ARE ESSENTIAL FOR MUSCLE RECOVERY AND GROWTH. INCORPORATE AT LEAST 2 REST DAYS PER WEEK IN YOUR WORKOUT SCHEDULE. THESE COULD BE COMPLETE REST OR ACTIVE RECOVERY DAYS.

SECTION 5.6: LISTENING TO YOUR BODY

IT'S ESSENTIAL TO LISTEN TO YOUR BODY AND RECOGNIZE SIGNS OF INADEQUATE RECOVERY, SUCH AS PERSISTENT FATIGUE, DECREASED PERFORMANCE, OR INCREASED INJURY RISK. IF YOU NOTICE THESE SIGNS, IT MIGHT BE TIME TO REASSESS YOUR RECOVERY STRATEGIES OR OVERALL WORKOUT ROUTINE.

SECTION 5.7: THE ROLE OF MOBILITY AND FLEXIBILITY EXERCISES

MOBILITY AND FLEXIBILITY EXERCISES, SUCH AS STRETCHING AND FOAM ROLLING, CAN ENHANCE MUSCLE RECOVERY BY IMPROVING BLOOD FLOW, REDUCING MUSCLE TENSION, AND INCREASING MUSCLE FLEXIBILITY.

RECOVERY IS A CRUCIAL BUT OFTEN OVERLOOKED COMPONENT OF MUSCLE GROWTH. BY PRIORITIZING RECOVERY – INCLUDING QUALITY SLEEP, ACTIVE RECOVERY, NUTRITION, HYDRATION, AND REST DAYS – YOU CAN ENSURE YOUR BODY EFFECTIVELY REPAIRS AND GROWS MUSCLE TISSUE. IN THE NEXT CHAPTER, WE WILL EXPLORE THE IMPORTANCE OF MENTAL FORTITUDE AND CONSISTENCY IN ACHIEVING SUSTAINABLE MUSCLE GROWTH. REMEMBER, MUSCLE BUILDING IS A MARATHON, NOT A SPRINT. BALANCING EXERCISE WITH ADEQUATE RECOVERY IS KEY TO LONG-TERM SUCCESS IN YOUR MUSCLE-BUILDING JOURNEY.

CHAPTER 6: MENTAL TOUGHNESS AND CONSISTENCY: THE KEY TO SUSTAINABLE GROWTH

THE PHYSICAL COMPONENTS OF MUSCLE GROWTH - WORKOUT, NUTRITION, AND RECOVERY - ARE UNDENIABLY IMPORTANT. HOWEVER, THE MENTAL ASPECT OF YOUR FITNESS JOURNEY IS EQUALLY CRITICAL. MENTAL TOUGHNESS AND CONSISTENCY FORM THE BACKBONE OF SUSTAINABLE GROWTH. IN THIS CHAPTER, WE EXPLORE THESE CRUCIAL COMPONENTS AND OFFER STRATEGIES TO CULTIVATE AND MAINTAIN THEM.

SECTION 6.1: THE ROLE OF MENTAL TOUGHNESS IN MUSCLE GROWTH

MENTAL TOUGHNESS, OR RESILIENCE, REFERS TO THE ABILITY TO REMAIN FOCUSED AND CONSISTENT, OVERCOME CHALLENGES, AND REBOUND FROM SETBACKS. BUILDING MUSCLE ISN'T JUST ABOUT THE BODY - IT'S A MENTAL GAME. STAYING MOTIVATED WHEN PROGRESS IS SLOW, PUSHING THROUGH TOUGH WORKOUTS, AND MAINTAINING DISCIPLINE WITH YOUR NUTRITION AND RECOVERY REQUIRE MENTAL STRENGTH AND DETERMINATION.

SECTION 6.2: STRATEGIES TO CULTIVATE MENTAL TOUGHNESS

HERE ARE SOME STRATEGIES TO CULTIVATE MENTAL TOUGHNESS:
1. SET CLEAR GOALS: HAVING SPECIFIC, MEASURABLE, ACHIEVABLE, RELEVANT, AND TIME-BOUND (SMART) GOALS CAN HELP KEEP YOU FOCUSED AND MOTIVATED.
2. POSITIVE SELF-TALK: POSITIVE SELF-TALK CAN HELP IMPROVE YOUR PERFORMANCE AND REDUCE THE PERCEPTION OF EXERTION.
3. MINDFULNESS AND MEDITATION: PRACTICES LIKE MINDFULNESS AND MEDITATION CAN ENHANCE YOUR MENTAL RESILIENCE, HELPING YOU STAY FOCUSED AND HANDLE STRESS MORE EFFECTIVELY.

SECTION 6.3: THE IMPORTANCE OF CONSISTENCY

CONSISTENCY IS ARGUABLY THE MOST CRITICAL FACTOR IN ACHIEVING SUSTAINABLE MUSCLE GROWTH. STICKING TO YOUR WORKOUT, NUTRITION, AND RECOVERY PLANS OVER THE LONG TERM IS WHAT LEADS TO NOTICEABLE CHANGES. IT'S ABOUT MAKING YOUR FITNESS ROUTINE A REGULAR PART OF YOUR LIFESTYLE.

SECTION 6.4: TIPS TO MAINTAIN CONSISTENCY

MAINTAINING CONSISTENCY CAN BE CHALLENGING, BUT THESE TIPS CAN HELP:
1. ESTABLISH A ROUTINE: HAVING A REGULAR WORKOUT SCHEDULE CAN HELP MAKE YOUR WORKOUTS A NONNEGOTIABLE PART OF YOUR DAY.
2. MIX THINGS UP: TO PREVENT BOREDOM AND PLATEAUING, REGULARLY CHANGE YOUR WORKOUT ROUTINE BY VARYING THE EXERCISES, INTENSITY, VOLUME, AND FREQUENCY.
3. TRACK YOUR PROGRESS: KEEPING A RECORD OF YOUR WORKOUTS AND PROGRESS CAN PROVIDE A SENSE OF ACHIEVEMENT AND HELP KEEP YOU MOTIVATED.

SECTION 6.5: DEALING WITH PLATEAUS

OVER TIME, YOU MAY HIT A PLATEAU WHERE PROGRESS SEEMS TO STALL. THIS IS A NORMAL PART OF THE MUSCLEBUILDING JOURNEY. WHEN THIS HAPPENS, CONSIDER ALTERING YOUR WORKOUT ROUTINE, REEVALUATING YOUR NUTRITION PLAN, OPTIMIZING YOUR RECOVERY, OR SEEKING ADVICE FROM A FITNESS PROFESSIONAL.
IN CONCLUSION, CULTIVATING MENTAL TOUGHNESS AND MAINTAINING CONSISTENCY ARE PIVOTAL TO ACHIEVING SUSTAINABLE MUSCLE GROWTH. REMEMBER, THE ROAD TO MUSCLE GROWTH ISN'T ALWAYS SMOOTH, BUT WITH RESILIENCE, DETERMINATION, AND CONSISTENCY, YOU CAN NAVIGATE THE CHALLENGES AND KEEP PROGRESSING TOWARDS YOUR FITNESS

GOALS. AS YOU EMBARK ON YOUR MUSCLE-BUILDING JOURNEY, ALWAYS REMEMBER - IT'S NOT JUST ABOUT THE DESTINATION BUT ALSO ABOUT THE JOURNEY. THE DISCIPLINE, RESILIENCE, AND CONSISTENCY YOU CULTIVATE ALONG THE WAY ARE REWARDS IN THEIR OWN RIGHT.

CHAPTER 7: THE CRUCIAL ROLE OF NUTRITION IN MAXIMUM MUSCLE GROWTH

THE JOURNEY TO MUSCLE GROWTH ISN'T CONFINED TO THE HOURS SPENT LIFTING WEIGHTS IN THE GYM. WHILE THE RIGHT TRAINING REGIMEN IS CRUCIAL, PROPER NUTRITION CAN SIGNIFICANTLY ENHANCE MUSCLE GROWTH, RECOVERY, AND OVERALL PHYSICAL PERFORMANCE. THIS CHAPTER EXPLORES THE VITAL ROLE OF NUTRITION IN MUSCLE GROWTH AND OFFERS GUIDELINES FOR FUELING YOUR BODY EFFECTIVELY FOR MAXIMUM GAINS.

SECTION 7.1: NUTRITION AND MUSCLE GROWTH - AN OVERVIEW

UNDERSTANDING THE IMPORTANCE OF NUTRITION IN MUSCLE GROWTH BEGINS WITH RECOGNIZING HOW MUSCLES GROW. WHEN WE WORK OUT, ESPECIALLY IN STRENGTH TRAINING, WE CREATE MICROSCOPIC TEARS IN OUR MUSCLE FIBERS. THE BODY REPAIRS THESE TEARS DURING REST PERIODS, LEADING TO AN INCREASE IN THE SIZE OF THE MUSCLE FIBERS, RESULTING IN MUSCLE GROWTH. HOWEVER, THIS REPAIR PROCESS REQUIRES NUTRIENTS - THE RAW MATERIALS FOR REPAIR AND GROWTH. INADEQUATE NUTRITION CAN HINDER MUSCLE RECOVERY AND GROWTH, DESPITE YOUR BEST WORKOUT EFFORTS.

SECTION 7.2: THE ROLE OF MACRONUTRIENTS

MACRONUTRIENTS - PROTEINS, CARBOHYDRATES, AND FATS - EACH PLAY SPECIFIC ROLES IN MUSCLE GROWTH:
1. PROTEIN: OFTEN TERMED THE BUILDING BLOCK OF MUSCLES, PROTEIN PROVIDES THE ESSENTIAL AMINO ACIDS NECESSARY FOR MUSCLE REPAIR AND GROWTH. CONSUMING ADEQUATE PROTEIN THROUGHOUT THE DAY ENSURES YOUR BODY HAS A STEADY SUPPLY OF AMINO ACIDS FOR MUSCLE PROTEIN SYNTHESIS.
2. CARBOHYDRATES: CARBS SERVE AS THE PRIMARY FUEL FOR YOUR WORKOUTS AND DAY-TO-DAY ACTIVITIES. THEY ALSO PLAY A CRUCIAL ROLE POST-WORKOUT BY REPLENISHING MUSCLE GLYCOGEN STORES, PROMOTING FASTER RECOVERY AND PREPARING YOUR MUSCLES FOR YOUR NEXT WORKOUT.
3. FATS: ALTHOUGH NOT DIRECTLY INVOLVED IN MUSCLE GROWTH, FATS SUPPORT OVERALL HEALTH, PROVIDE ENERGY, AND AID IN THE ABSORPTION OF CERTAIN VITAMINS. HEALTHY FATS ALSO PLAY A KEY ROLE IN MAINTAINING OPTIMAL HORMONE LEVELS, INCLUDING TESTOSTERONE, WHICH IS IMPORTANT FOR MUSCLE GROWTH.

SECTION 7.3: THE SIGNIFICANCE OF MICRONUTRIENTS AND HYDRATION

MICRONUTRIENTS, INCLUDING VITAMINS AND MINERALS, SUPPORT VARIOUS BODILY FUNCTIONS, INCLUDING ENERGY PRODUCTION, BONE HEALTH, AND IMMUNE FUNCTION. STAYING HYDRATED IS ALSO VITAL AS WATER PLAYS A ROLE IN VIRTUALLY ALL BODILY FUNCTIONS, INCLUDING NUTRIENT TRANSPORT AND MUSCLE CONTRACTION.

SECTION 7.4: NUTRIENT TIMING FOR MUSCLE GROWTH

WHILE IT'S IMPORTANT WHAT YOU EAT, WHEN YOU EAT CAN ALSO IMPACT MUSCLE GROWTH. CONSUMING A BALANCED MEAL OR SNACK CONTAINING PROTEIN AND CARBOHYDRATES POST-WORKOUT CAN MAXIMIZE MUSCLE PROTEIN SYNTHESIS AND RECOVERY.

SECTION 7.5: CUSTOMIZING YOUR NUTRITION PLAN

NUTRITIONAL NEEDS CAN VARY WIDELY BASED ON FACTORS LIKE AGE, GENDER, WEIGHT, TRAINING INTENSITY, AND MUSCLE GROWTH GOALS. THEREFORE, IT'S IMPORTANT TO PERSONALIZE YOUR NUTRITION PLAN TO BEST SUPPORT YOUR MUSCLE GROWTH JOURNEY.

IN SUMMARY, PROPER NUTRITION IS A POWERFUL TOOL THAT WORKS HAND IN HAND WITH YOUR WORKOUT REGIMEN TO MAXIMIZE MUSCLE GROWTH. BY UNDERSTANDING AND APPLYING THE PRINCIPLES OF NUTRITION, YOU CAN FUEL YOUR BODY EFFECTIVELY TO SUPPORT MUSCLE REPAIR, RECOVERY, AND GROWTH. REMEMBER, EVERY STEP YOU TAKE TOWARDS BETTER NUTRITION IS A STEP TOWARDS MAXIMIZING YOUR MUSCLE GROWTH POTENTIAL. NUTRITION IN ITSELF IS A WHOLE OTHER TOPIC THAT WE CAN SPEND HOURS AND A WHOLE OTHER BOOK DISCUSSION, BUT FOR THE SAKE OF BREVITY I HAVE SIMPLIFIED THIS TOPIC AND GIVEN YOU A QUICK OVERVIEW OF THE BASICS OF NUTRITION, IN A FOLLOW UP SERIES, WE WILL DELVE DEEPER INTO THE TOPIC OF PROPER NUTRITION FOR STRENGTH TRAINING AND MUSCLE-BUILDING.

CONCLUSION: ACHIEVING MAXIMUM MUSCLE GROWTH - THE ROAD AHEAD

AS WE DRAW THIS GUIDE TO A CLOSE, IT'S IMPORTANT TO REMEMBER THAT THE ROAD TO MAXIMUM MUSCLE GROWTH ISN'T A STRAIGHTFORWARD ONE, BUT RATHER A JOURNEY. IT'S A JOURNEY OF UNDERSTANDING THE INTRICATE WORKINGS OF YOUR BODY, FUELING IT WITH THE RIGHT NUTRIENTS, PUSHING IT BEYOND ITS COMFORT ZONE, AND GIVING IT THE REST IT NEEDS TO REPAIR AND GROW STRONGER. WE HAVE EXPLORED THE SCIENCE BEHIND MUSCLE GROWTH, SHEDDING LIGHT ON THE ROLE OF MUSCLE FIBERS, HORMONES, AND THE PROCESS OF MUSCLE PROTEIN SYNTHESIS. THIS KNOWLEDGE SETS THE STAGE FOR UNDERSTANDING
WHY CERTAIN WORKOUT ROUTINES AND DIETARY CHOICES CAN MAXIMIZE MUSCLE GROWTH. WE DELVED INTO THE CRUCIAL ROLE OF NUTRITION, COVERING THE IMPORTANCE OF MACRONUTRIENTS - PROTEIN, CARBOHYDRATES, AND FATS - AS WELL AS MICRONUTRIENTS AND HYDRATION. WE'VE ESTABLISHED THAT WHILE WHAT WE EAT PLAYS A SIGNIFICANT ROLE, WHEN WE EAT, PARTICULARLY AROUND OUR WORKOUTS, CAN ALSO INFLUENCE MUSCLE GROWTH. NEXT, WE JOURNEYED THROUGH THE PROCESS OF DESIGNING A MUSCLE-BUILDING WORKOUT REGIME, FOCUSING ON THE PRINCIPLES OF EXERCISE SELECTION, VOLUME, INTENSITY, AND FREQUENCY. WE ALSO OUTLINED HOW TO BALANCE WORKOUTS TO AVOID IMBALANCES AND THE IMPORTANCE OF THE PRINCIPLE OF PROGRESSIVE OVERLOAD FOR CONTINUOUS GROWTH. WE PROVIDED DETAILED WORKOUT PROGRAMS TO CATER TO DIFFERENT FITNESS LEVELS, FROM BEGINNERS JUST EMBARKING ON THEIR MUSCLE-BUILDING JOURNEY TO ADVANCED FITNESS ENTHUSIASTS LOOKING TO PUSH THEIR BOUNDARIES.
WE THEN TURNED OUR ATTENTION TO THE OFTEN OVERLOOKED YET ESSENTIAL COMPONENT OF MUSCLE GROWTH - RECOVERY.

EMPHASIZING THE ROLE OF QUALITY SLEEP, ACTIVE RECOVERY, NUTRITION, HYDRATION, AND REST DAYS, WE UNDERSCORED THAT RECOVERY IS WHEN THE ACTUAL GROWTH HAPPENS. FINALLY, WE EXPLORED THE MENTAL ASPECT OF MUSCLE GROWTH, DISCUSSING THE IMPORTANCE OF MENTAL TOUGHNESS AND CONSISTENCY. THESE ASPECTS ARE WHAT KEEP YOU SHOWING UP, PUSHING THROUGH, AND COMING BACK, EVEN
WHEN PROGRESS SEEMS SLOW. IT'S IMPORTANT TO REMEMBER THAT WHILE THIS GUIDE PROVIDES A ROADMAP TO MUSCLE GROWTH, EACH PERSON'S
JOURNEY IS UNIQUE. OUR BODIES RESPOND DIFFERENTLY TO WORKOUTS AND NUTRITION. LISTENING TO YOUR BODY, BEING PATIENT WITH THE PROCESS, AND MAKING ADJUSTMENTS AS NEEDED IS KEY. REMEMBER, THE PURSUIT OF MUSCLE GROWTH IS MORE THAN JUST ABOUT AESTHETICS OR STRENGTH. IT'S A COMMITMENT TO YOUR HEALTH, DISCIPLINE, AND PERSONAL GROWTH. IT'S ABOUT SETTING GOALS AND WORKING TOWARDS THEM, OVERCOMING CHALLENGES ALONG THE WAY, AND BECOMING THE BEST VERSION OF YOURSELF.

WE HOPE THIS GUIDE EQUIPS YOU WITH THE KNOWLEDGE AND TOOLS TO NAVIGATE YOUR MUSCLE-BUILDING JOURNEY EFFECTIVELY. HERE'S TO YOUR SUCCESS IN ACHIEVING MAXIMUM MUSCLE GROWTH AND THE MANY REWARDS THAT COME ALONG WITH IT!

ILLUSTRATIONS

Leg Exercises

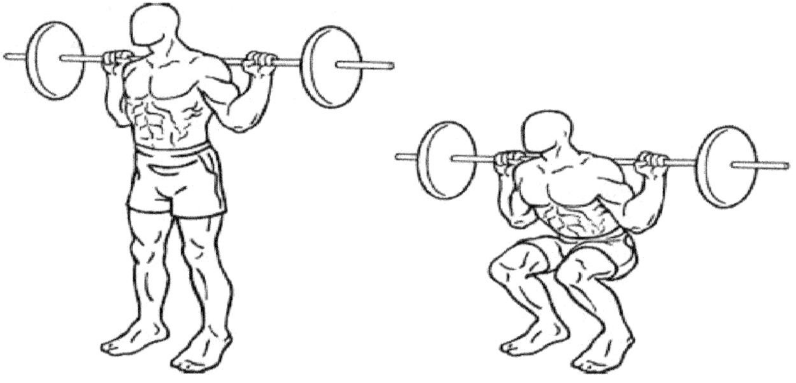

Squats

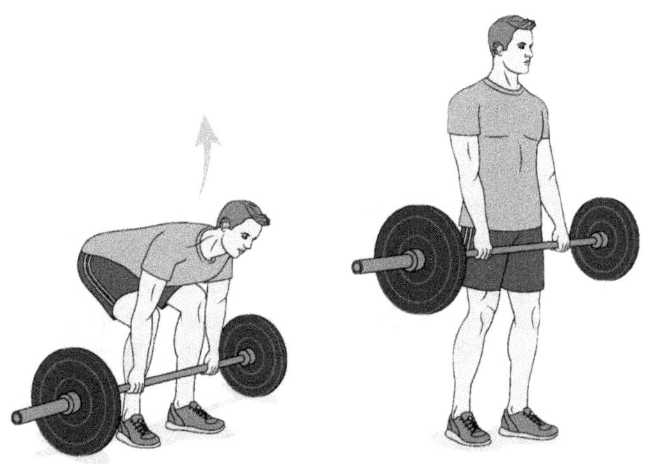

Deadlifts

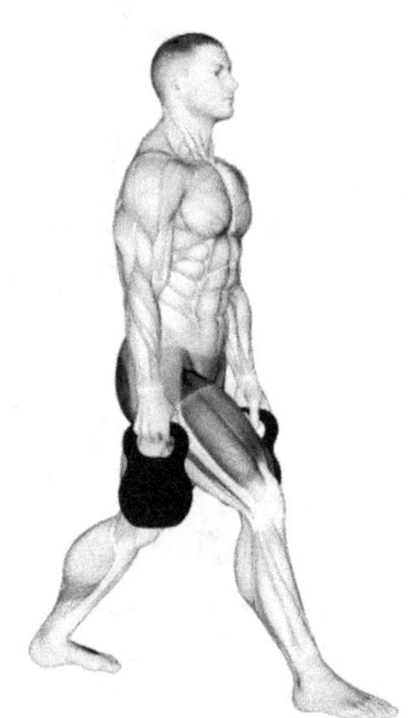
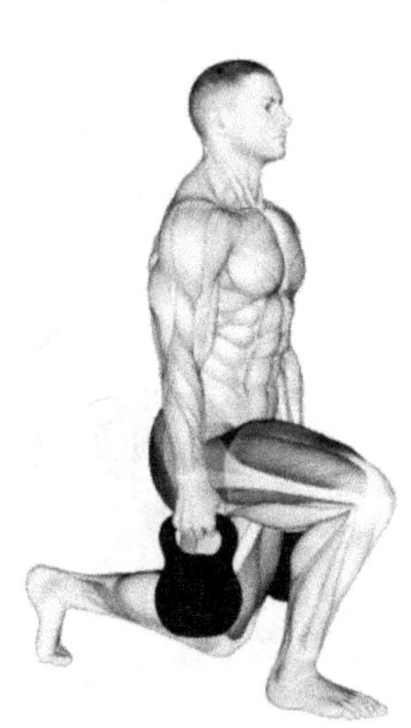

Lunges

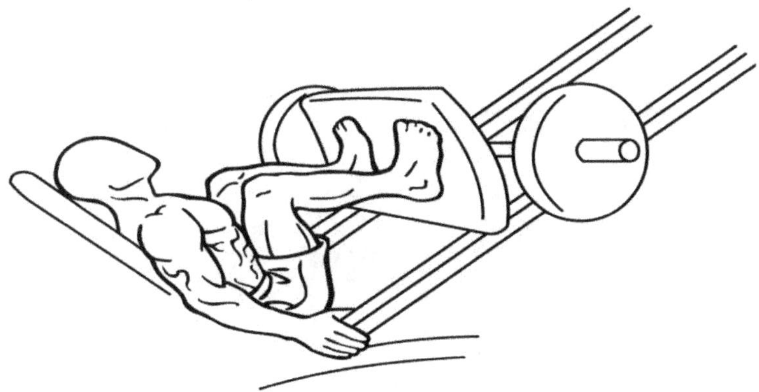

Leg Press

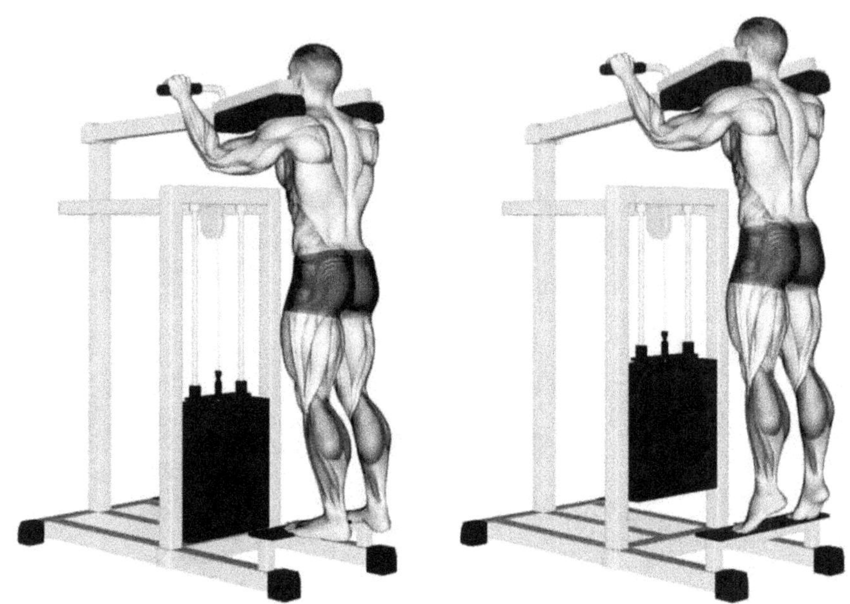

Calf Raises

Back Exercises

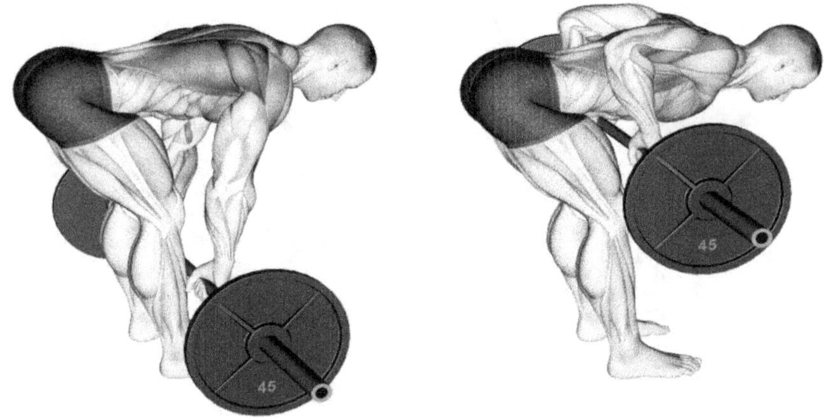

Bent Over Rows

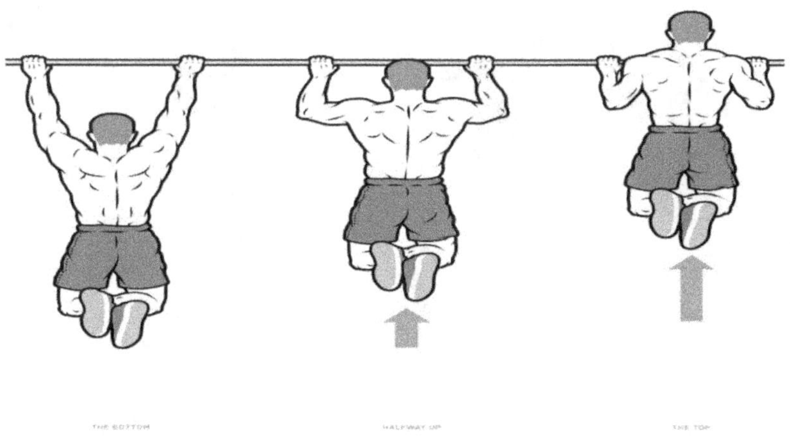

Pull Ups

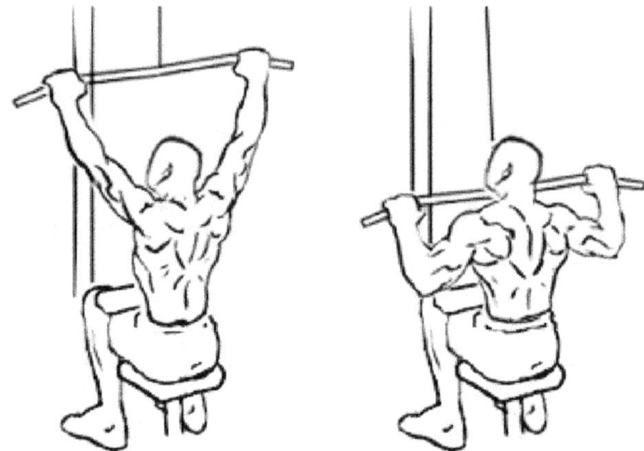

Latt Pulldown

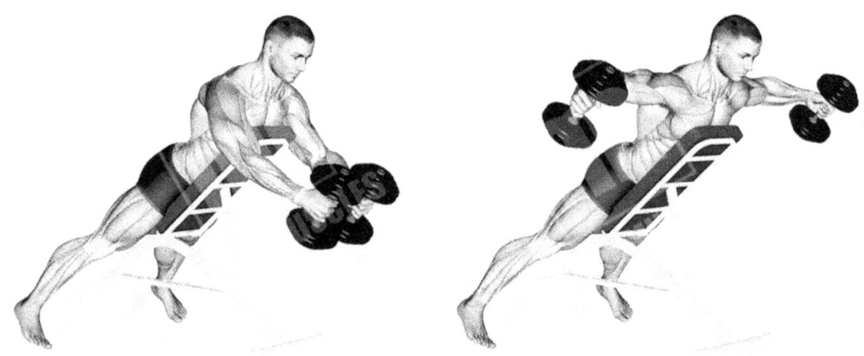

Rear Delt Flyes

Chest Exercises

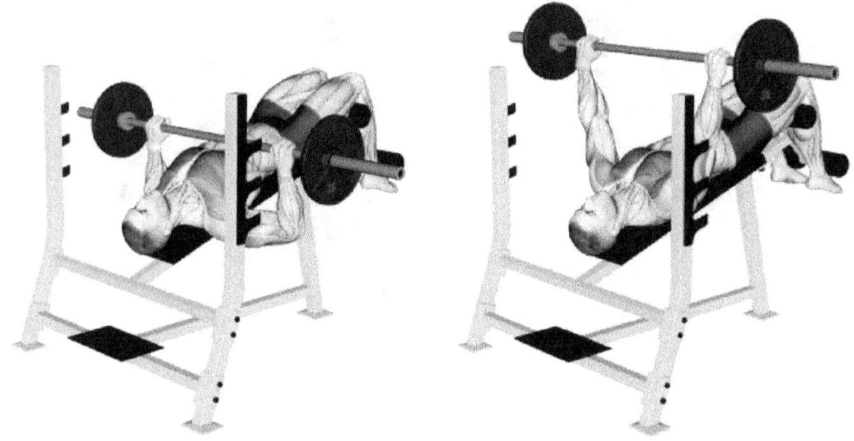

Decline Bench Press

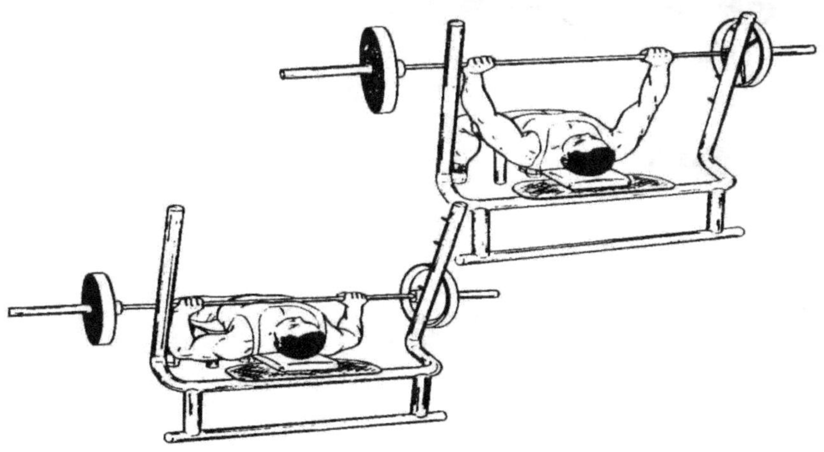

Bench Press

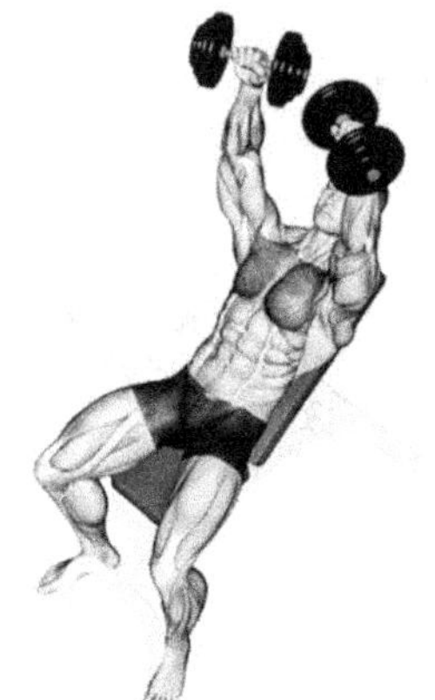 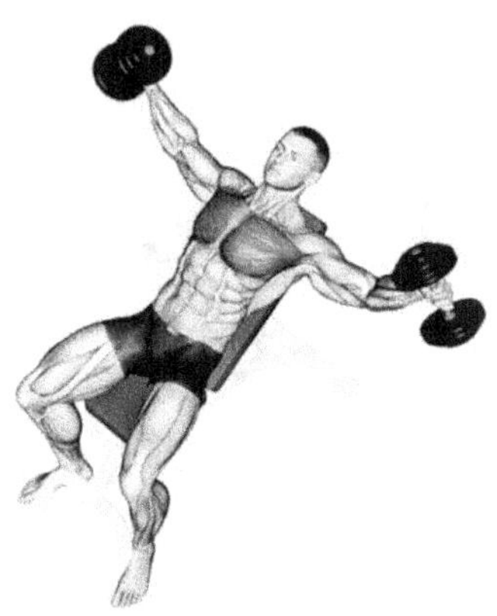

Dumbbell Flyes

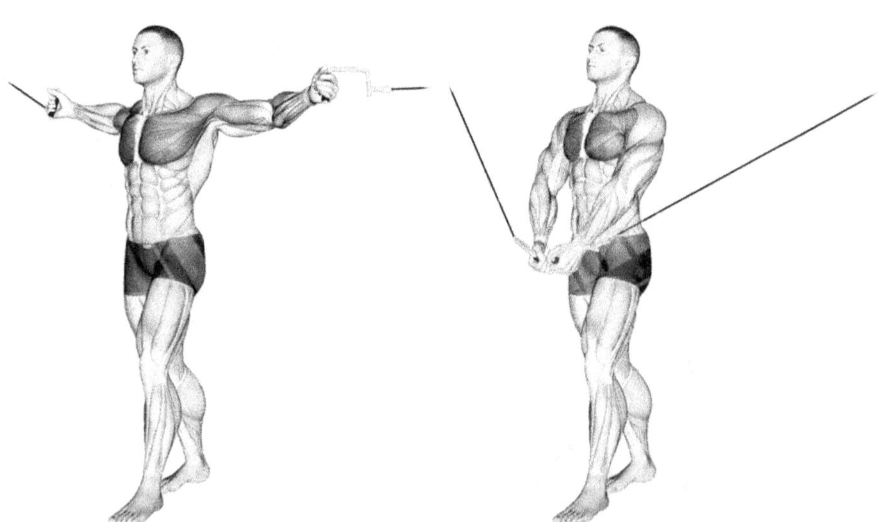

Cable Crossovers

Shoulder Exercises

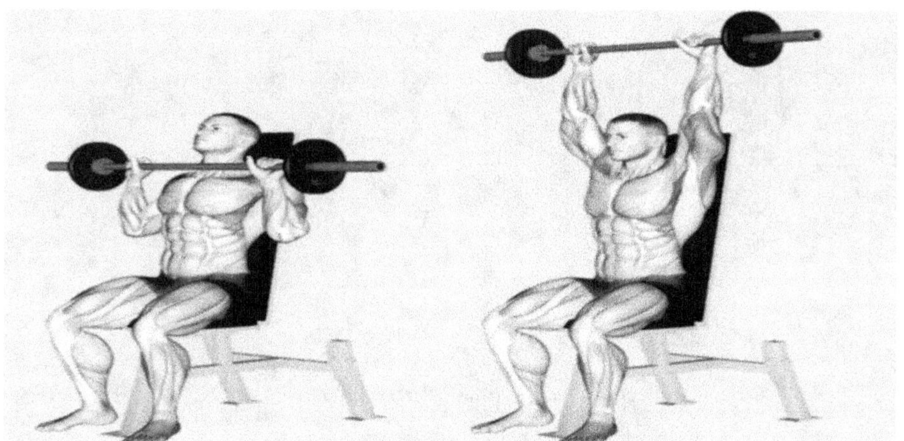

Overhead Press

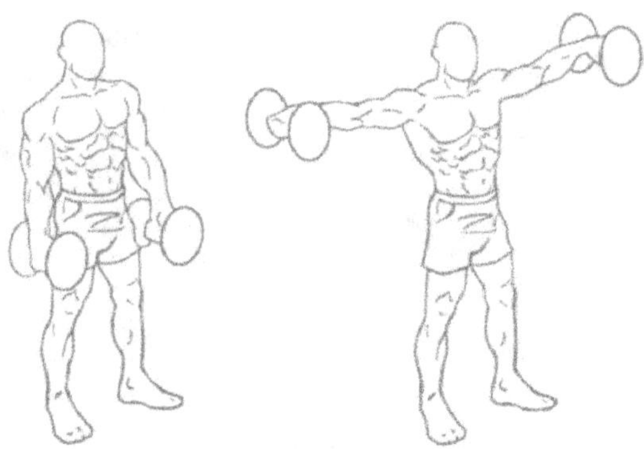

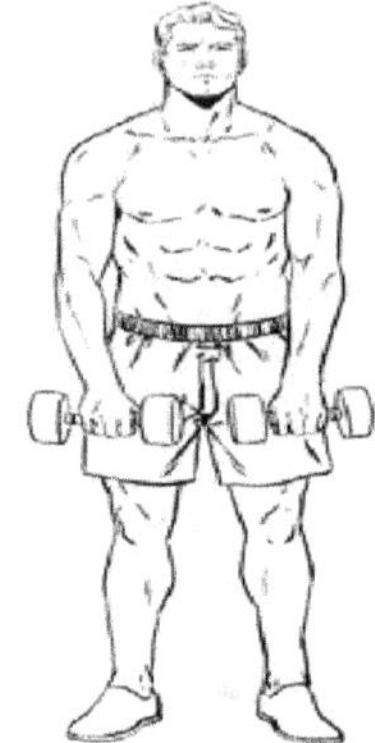 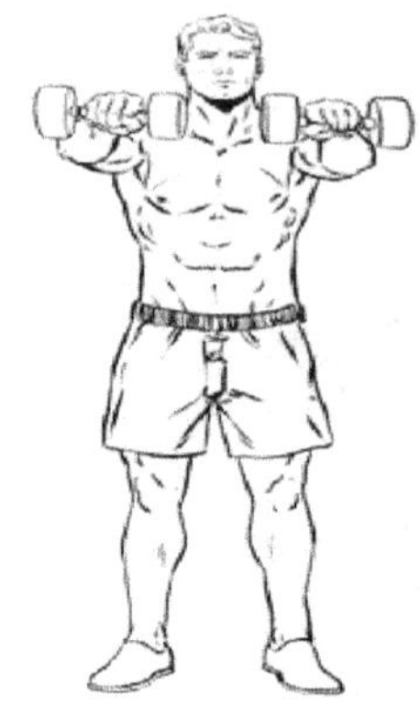

Front Dumbbell Raises

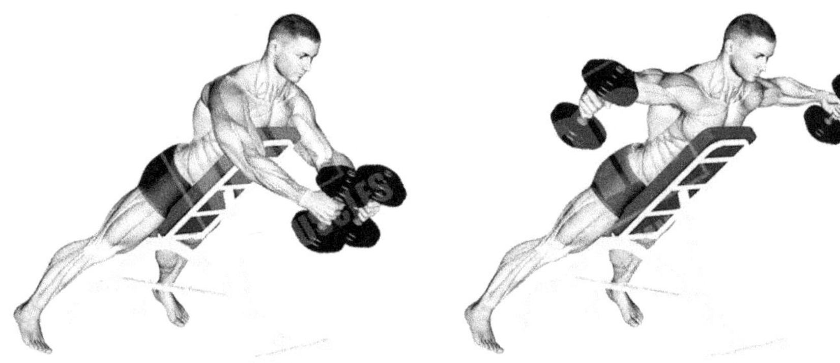

Rear Delt Flyes

Arm Exercises

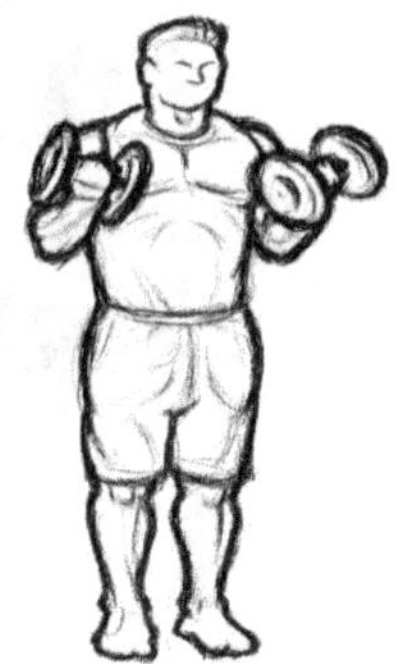

Bicep Curls

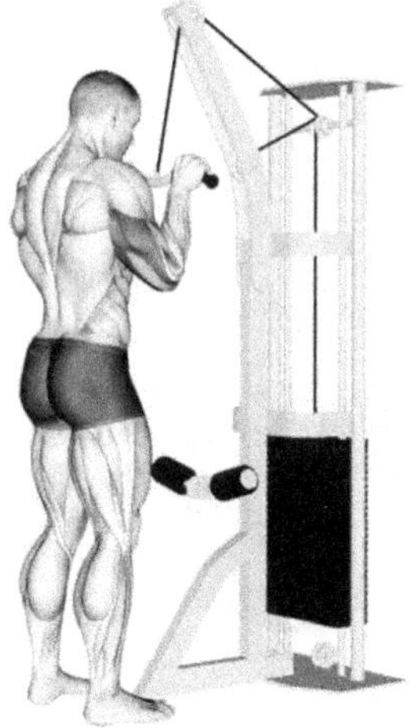 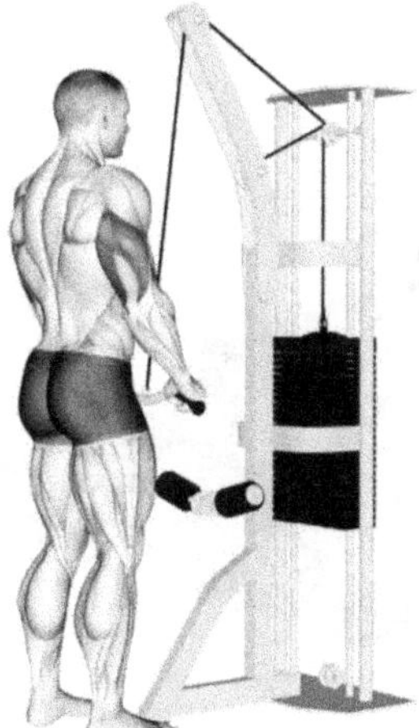

Tricep Pushdowns

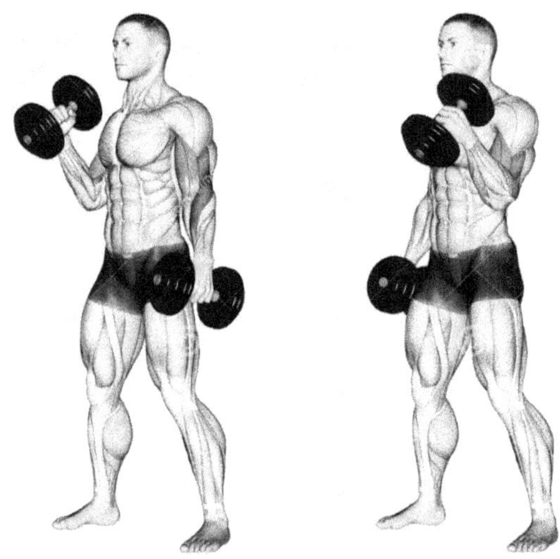

Dumbbell Hammer Curls

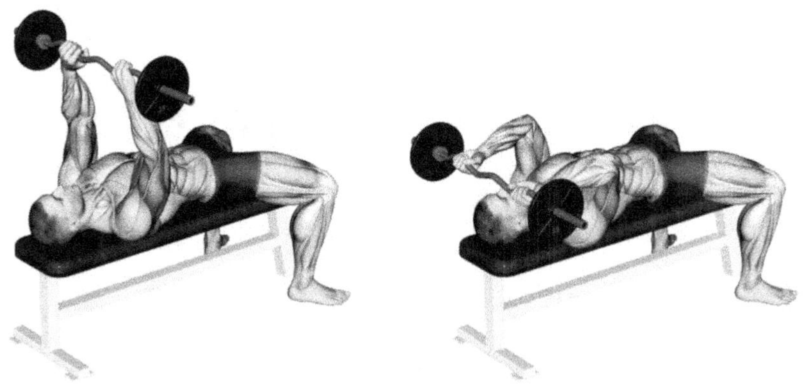

Skull Crushers

Core Exercises

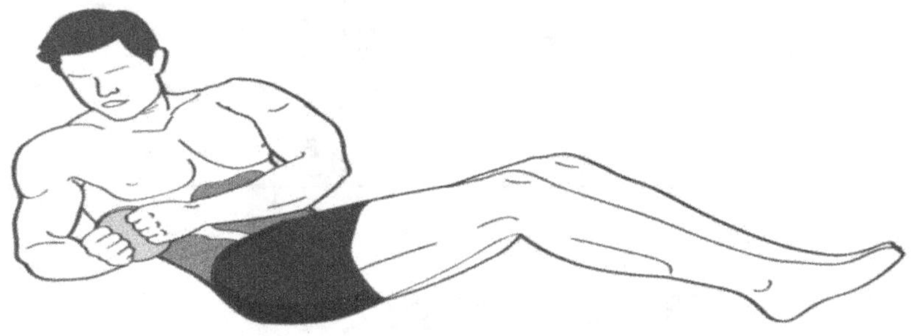

Russian Twists

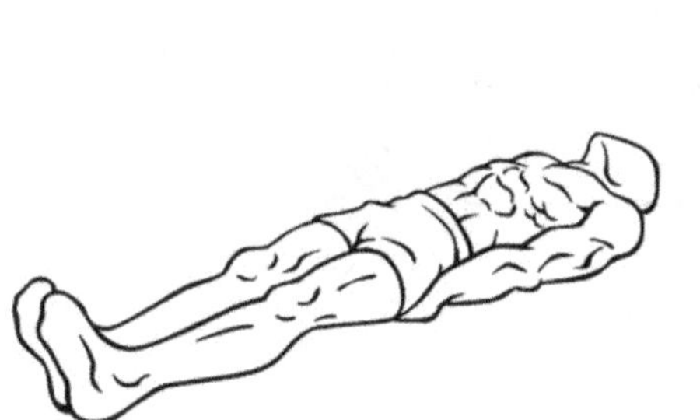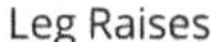

Leg Raises

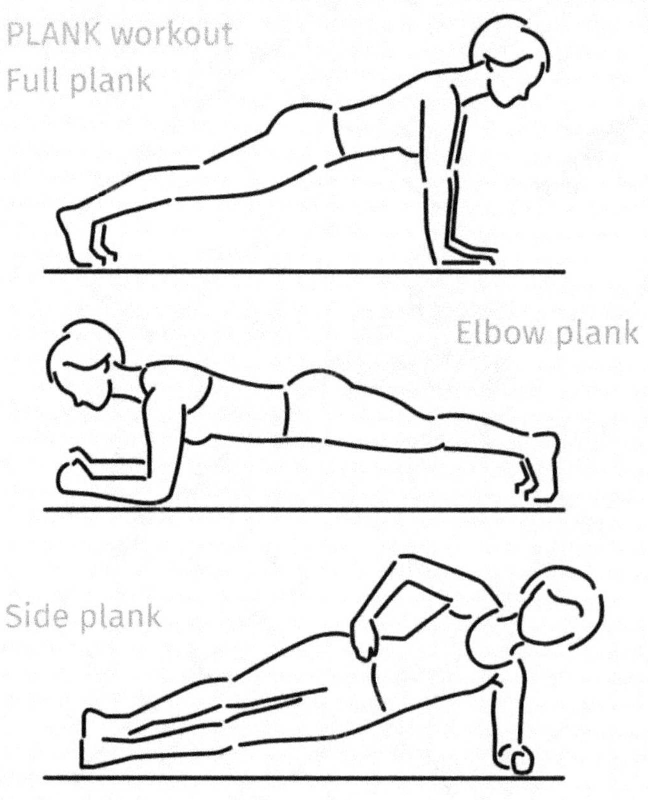

Planks